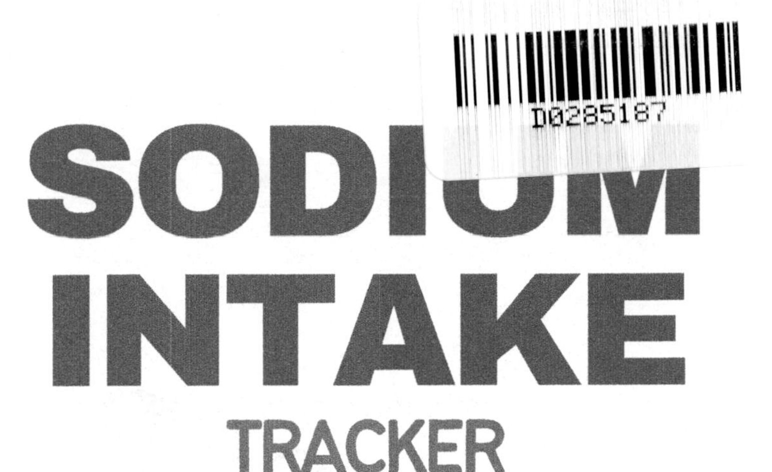
D0285187
INTAKE
TRACKER

SODIUM TRACKER

DAILY SODIUM INTAKE GOAL : 2,300 mg

DATE : Apr 22, 2022

	FOOD & DRINKS	SERVING SIZE	SODIUM	SYMPTOMS/NOTES
BREAKFAST	Fried eggs	2	95 mg	
	Toast with butter	1	173 mg	
	coffee	1 cup	15 mg	made at home, no cream & sugar
SNACK	low fat blueberry muffin	1	410 mg	
LUNCH	Chicken sandwich		160 mg	whole meal bread and 40 g steam chicken
	Steamed broccoli	2 cups	30 mg	no salt added
	Diet soda	12 fl oz	28 mg	mild bloating
SNACK	Lay's potato chips	1 oz	170 mg	snack eaten to improve nausea symptoms
	Electrolyte drink	8 fl oz	95 mg	
DINNER	Vegetarian pizza	3 slices	1,320 mg	mild bloating and abdominal pain after eating
	Garden salad with dressing		250 mg	1 tbsp Italian dressing
	DAILY SODIUM TOTAL		2,841 mg	

NOTES : I exceeded my sodium intake goal for the day. ☹ Tomorrow, I'm going to try to limit my salt intake!

SODIUM TRACKER

DAILY SODIUM INTAKE GOAL :

DATE :

	FOOD & DRINKS	SERVING SIZE	SODIUM	SYMPTOMS / NOTES
BREAKFAST				
SNACK				
LUNCH				
SNACK				
DINNER				
	DAILY SODIUM TOTAL			

NOTES :

SODIUM TRACKER

DAILY SODIUM INTAKE GOAL :

DATE :

	FOOD & DRINKS	SERVING SIZE	SODIUM	SYMPTOMS / NOTES
BREAKFAST				
SNACK				
LUNCH				
SNACK				
DINNER				
	DAILY SODIUM TOTAL			

NOTES :

SODIUM TRACKER

DAILY SODIUM INTAKE GOAL :

DATE :

	FOOD & DRINKS	SERVING SIZE	SODIUM	SYMPTOMS / NOTES
BREAKFAST				
SNACK				
LUNCH				
SNACK				
DINNER				
	DAILY SODIUM TOTAL			

NOTES :

SODIUM TRACKER

DAILY SODIUM INTAKE GOAL :

DATE :

	FOOD & DRINKS	SERVING SIZE	SODIUM	SYMPTOMS / NOTES
BREAKFAST				
SNACK				
LUNCH				
SNACK				
DINNER				
	DAILY SODIUM TOTAL			

NOTES :

SODIUM TRACKER

DAILY SODIUM INTAKE GOAL :

DATE :

	FOOD & DRINKS	SERVING SIZE	SODIUM	SYMPTOMS / NOTES
BREAKFAST				
SNACK				
LUNCH				
SNACK				
DINNER				
	DAILY SODIUM TOTAL			

NOTES :

SODIUM TRACKER

DAILY SODIUM INTAKE GOAL :

DATE :

	FOOD & DRINKS	SERVING SIZE	SODIUM	SYMPTOMS / NOTES
BREAKFAST				
SNACK				
LUNCH				
SNACK				
DINNER				
	DAILY SODIUM TOTAL			

NOTES :

SODIUM TRACKER

DAILY SODIUM INTAKE GOAL :

DATE :

	FOOD & DRINKS	SERVING SIZE	SODIUM	SYMPTOMS / NOTES
BREAKFAST				
SNACK				
LUNCH				
SNACK				
DINNER				
	DAILY SODIUM TOTAL			

NOTES :

SODIUM TRACKER

DAILY SODIUM INTAKE GOAL :

DATE :

	FOOD & DRINKS	SERVING SIZE	SODIUM	SYMPTOMS / NOTES
BREAKFAST				
SNACK				
LUNCH				
SNACK				
DINNER				
	DAILY SODIUM TOTAL			

NOTES :

SODIUM TRACKER

DAILY SODIUM INTAKE GOAL :

DATE :

	FOOD & DRINKS	SERVING SIZE	SODIUM	SYMPTOMS / NOTES
BREAKFAST				
SNACK				
LUNCH				
SNACK				
DINNER				
	DAILY SODIUM TOTAL			

NOTES :

SODIUM TRACKER

DAILY SODIUM INTAKE GOAL :

DATE :

	FOOD & DRINKS	SERVING SIZE	SODIUM	SYMPTOMS / NOTES
BREAKFAST				
SNACK				
LUNCH				
SNACK				
DINNER				
	DAILY SODIUM TOTAL			

NOTES :

SODIUM TRACKER

DAILY SODIUM INTAKE GOAL :

DATE :

	FOOD & DRINKS	SERVING SIZE	SODIUM	SYMPTOMS / NOTES
BREAKFAST				
SNACK				
LUNCH				
SNACK				
DINNER				
	DAILY SODIUM TOTAL			

NOTES :

SODIUM TRACKER

DAILY SODIUM INTAKE GOAL :

DATE :

	FOOD & DRINKS	SERVING SIZE	SODIUM	SYMPTOMS / NOTES
BREAKFAST				
SNACK				
LUNCH				
SNACK				
DINNER				
	DAILY SODIUM TOTAL			

NOTES :

SODIUM TRACKER

DAILY SODIUM INTAKE GOAL :

DATE :

	FOOD & DRINKS	SERVING SIZE	SODIUM	SYMPTOMS / NOTES
BREAKFAST				
SNACK				
LUNCH				
SNACK				
DINNER				
	DAILY SODIUM TOTAL			

NOTES :

SODIUM TRACKER

DAILY SODIUM INTAKE GOAL :

DATE :

	FOOD & DRINKS	SERVING SIZE	SODIUM	SYMPTOMS / NOTES
BREAKFAST				
SNACK				
LUNCH				
SNACK				
DINNER				
	DAILY SODIUM TOTAL			

NOTES :

SODIUM TRACKER

DAILY SODIUM INTAKE GOAL :

DATE :

	FOOD & DRINKS	SERVING SIZE	SODIUM	SYMPTOMS / NOTES
BREAKFAST				
SNACK				
LUNCH				
SNACK				
DINNER				
	DAILY SODIUM TOTAL			

NOTES :

SODIUM TRACKER

DAILY SODIUM INTAKE GOAL :

DATE :

	FOOD & DRINKS	SERVING SIZE	SODIUM	SYMPTOMS / NOTES
BREAKFAST				
SNACK				
LUNCH				
SNACK				
DINNER				
	DAILY SODIUM TOTAL			

NOTES :

SODIUM TRACKER

DAILY SODIUM INTAKE GOAL :

DATE :

	FOOD & DRINKS	SERVING SIZE	SODIUM	SYMPTOMS / NOTES
BREAKFAST				
SNACK				
LUNCH				
SNACK				
DINNER				
	DAILY SODIUM TOTAL			

NOTES :

SODIUM TRACKER

DAILY SODIUM INTAKE GOAL :

DATE :

	FOOD & DRINKS	SERVING SIZE	SODIUM	SYMPTOMS / NOTES
BREAKFAST				
SNACK				
LUNCH				
SNACK				
DINNER				
	DAILY SODIUM TOTAL			

NOTES :

SODIUM TRACKER

DAILY SODIUM INTAKE GOAL :

DATE :

	FOOD & DRINKS	SERVING SIZE	SODIUM	SYMPTOMS / NOTES
BREAKFAST				
SNACK				
LUNCH				
SNACK				
DINNER				
	DAILY SODIUM TOTAL			

NOTES :

SODIUM TRACKER

DAILY SODIUM INTAKE GOAL :

DATE :

	FOOD & DRINKS	SERVING SIZE	SODIUM	SYMPTOMS / NOTES
BREAKFAST				
SNACK				
LUNCH				
SNACK				
DINNER				
	DAILY SODIUM TOTAL			

NOTES :

SODIUM TRACKER

DAILY SODIUM INTAKE GOAL :	DATE :

	FOOD & DRINKS	SERVING SIZE	SODIUM	SYMPTOMS / NOTES
BREAKFAST				
SNACK				
LUNCH				
SNACK				
DINNER				
	DAILY SODIUM TOTAL			

NOTES :

SODIUM TRACKER

DAILY SODIUM INTAKE GOAL :

DATE :

	FOOD & DRINKS	SERVING SIZE	SODIUM	SYMPTOMS / NOTES
BREAKFAST				
SNACK				
LUNCH				
SNACK				
DINNER				
	DAILY SODIUM TOTAL			

NOTES :

SODIUM TRACKER

DAILY SODIUM INTAKE GOAL :

DATE :

	FOOD & DRINKS	SERVING SIZE	SODIUM	SYMPTOMS / NOTES
BREAKFAST				
SNACK				
LUNCH				
SNACK				
DINNER				
	DAILY SODIUM TOTAL			

NOTES :

SODIUM TRACKER

DAILY SODIUM INTAKE GOAL :

DATE :

	FOOD & DRINKS	SERVING SIZE	SODIUM	SYMPTOMS / NOTES
BREAKFAST				
SNACK				
LUNCH				
SNACK				
DINNER				
	DAILY SODIUM TOTAL			

NOTES :

SODIUM TRACKER

DAILY SODIUM INTAKE GOAL :

DATE :

	FOOD & DRINKS	SERVING SIZE	SODIUM	SYMPTOMS / NOTES
BREAKFAST				
SNACK				
LUNCH				
SNACK				
DINNER				
	DAILY SODIUM TOTAL			

NOTES :

SODIUM TRACKER

DAILY SODIUM INTAKE GOAL :

DATE :

	FOOD & DRINKS	SERVING SIZE	SODIUM	SYMPTOMS / NOTES
BREAKFAST				
SNACK				
LUNCH				
SNACK				
DINNER				
	DAILY SODIUM TOTAL			

NOTES :

SODIUM TRACKER

DAILY SODIUM INTAKE GOAL :

DATE :

	FOOD & DRINKS	SERVING SIZE	SODIUM	SYMPTOMS / NOTES
BREAKFAST				
SNACK				
LUNCH				
SNACK				
DINNER				
	DAILY SODIUM TOTAL			

NOTES :

SODIUM TRACKER

DAILY SODIUM INTAKE GOAL :

DATE :

	FOOD & DRINKS	SERVING SIZE	SODIUM	SYMPTOMS / NOTES
BREAKFAST				
SNACK				
LUNCH				
SNACK				
DINNER				
	DAILY SODIUM TOTAL			

NOTES :

SODIUM TRACKER

DAILY SODIUM INTAKE GOAL :

DATE :

	FOOD & DRINKS	SERVING SIZE	SODIUM	SYMPTOMS / NOTES
BREAKFAST				
SNACK				
LUNCH				
SNACK				
DINNER				
	DAILY SODIUM TOTAL			

NOTES :

SODIUM TRACKER

DAILY SODIUM INTAKE GOAL :

DATE :

	FOOD & DRINKS	SERVING SIZE	SODIUM	SYMPTOMS / NOTES
BREAKFAST				
SNACK				
LUNCH				
SNACK				
DINNER				
	DAILY SODIUM TOTAL			

NOTES :

SODIUM TRACKER

DAILY SODIUM INTAKE GOAL :

DATE :

	FOOD & DRINKS	SERVING SIZE	SODIUM	SYMPTOMS / NOTES
BREAKFAST				
SNACK				
LUNCH				
SNACK				
DINNER				
	DAILY SODIUM TOTAL			

NOTES :

SODIUM TRACKER

DAILY SODIUM INTAKE GOAL :

DATE :

	FOOD & DRINKS	SERVING SIZE	SODIUM	SYMPTOMS / NOTES
BREAKFAST				
SNACK				
LUNCH				
SNACK				
DINNER				
	DAILY SODIUM TOTAL			

NOTES :

SODIUM TRACKER

DAILY SODIUM INTAKE GOAL :	DATE :

	FOOD & DRINKS	SERVING SIZE	SODIUM	SYMPTOMS / NOTES
BREAKFAST				
SNACK				
LUNCH				
SNACK				
DINNER				
	DAILY SODIUM TOTAL			

NOTES :

SODIUM TRACKER

DAILY SODIUM INTAKE GOAL :

DATE :

	FOOD & DRINKS	SERVING SIZE	SODIUM	SYMPTOMS / NOTES
BREAKFAST				
SNACK				
LUNCH				
SNACK				
DINNER				
	DAILY SODIUM TOTAL			

NOTES :

SODIUM TRACKER

DAILY SODIUM INTAKE GOAL :

DATE :

	FOOD & DRINKS	SERVING SIZE	SODIUM	SYMPTOMS / NOTES
BREAKFAST				
SNACK				
LUNCH				
SNACK				
DINNER				
	DAILY SODIUM TOTAL			

NOTES :

SODIUM TRACKER

DAILY SODIUM INTAKE GOAL :

DATE :

	FOOD & DRINKS	SERVING SIZE	SODIUM	SYMPTOMS / NOTES
BREAKFAST				
SNACK				
LUNCH				
SNACK				
DINNER				
	DAILY SODIUM TOTAL			

NOTES :

SODIUM TRACKER

DAILY SODIUM INTAKE GOAL :

DATE :

	FOOD & DRINKS	SERVING SIZE	SODIUM	SYMPTOMS / NOTES
BREAKFAST				
SNACK				
LUNCH				
SNACK				
DINNER				
	DAILY SODIUM TOTAL			

NOTES :

SODIUM TRACKER

DAILY SODIUM INTAKE GOAL :

DATE :

	FOOD & DRINKS	SERVING SIZE	SODIUM	SYMPTOMS / NOTES
BREAKFAST				
SNACK				
LUNCH				
SNACK				
DINNER				
	DAILY SODIUM TOTAL			

NOTES :

SODIUM TRACKER

DAILY SODIUM INTAKE GOAL :

DATE :

	FOOD & DRINKS	SERVING SIZE	SODIUM	SYMPTOMS / NOTES
BREAKFAST				
SNACK				
LUNCH				
SNACK				
DINNER				
	DAILY SODIUM TOTAL			

NOTES :

SODIUM TRACKER

DAILY SODIUM INTAKE GOAL :

DATE :

	FOOD & DRINKS	SERVING SIZE	SODIUM	SYMPTOMS / NOTES
BREAKFAST				
SNACK				
LUNCH				
SNACK				
DINNER				
	DAILY SODIUM TOTAL			

NOTES :

SODIUM TRACKER

DAILY SODIUM INTAKE GOAL :

DATE :

	FOOD & DRINKS	SERVING SIZE	SODIUM	SYMPTOMS / NOTES
BREAKFAST				
SNACK				
LUNCH				
SNACK				
DINNER				
	DAILY SODIUM TOTAL			

NOTES :

SODIUM TRACKER

DAILY SODIUM INTAKE GOAL :

DATE :

	FOOD & DRINKS	SERVING SIZE	SODIUM	SYMPTOMS / NOTES
BREAKFAST				
SNACK				
LUNCH				
SNACK				
DINNER				
	DAILY SODIUM TOTAL			

NOTES :

SODIUM TRACKER

DAILY SODIUM INTAKE GOAL :

DATE :

	FOOD & DRINKS	SERVING SIZE	SODIUM	SYMPTOMS / NOTES
BREAKFAST				
SNACK				
LUNCH				
SNACK				
DINNER				
	DAILY SODIUM TOTAL			

NOTES :

SODIUM TRACKER

DAILY SODIUM INTAKE GOAL :

DATE :

	FOOD & DRINKS	SERVING SIZE	SODIUM	SYMPTOMS / NOTES
BREAKFAST				
SNACK				
LUNCH				
SNACK				
DINNER				
	DAILY SODIUM TOTAL			

NOTES :

SODIUM TRACKER

DAILY SODIUM INTAKE GOAL :

DATE :

	FOOD & DRINKS	SERVING SIZE	SODIUM	SYMPTOMS / NOTES
BREAKFAST				
SNACK				
LUNCH				
SNACK				
DINNER				
	DAILY SODIUM TOTAL			

NOTES :

SODIUM TRACKER

DAILY SODIUM INTAKE GOAL :	DATE :

	FOOD & DRINKS	SERVING SIZE	SODIUM	SYMPTOMS / NOTES
BREAKFAST				
SNACK				
LUNCH				
SNACK				
DINNER				
	DAILY SODIUM TOTAL			

NOTES :

SODIUM TRACKER

DAILY SODIUM INTAKE GOAL :

DATE :

	FOOD & DRINKS	SERVING SIZE	SODIUM	SYMPTOMS / NOTES
BREAKFAST				
SNACK				
LUNCH				
SNACK				
DINNER				
	DAILY SODIUM TOTAL			

NOTES :

SODIUM TRACKER

DAILY SODIUM INTAKE GOAL :

DATE :

	FOOD & DRINKS	SERVING SIZE	SODIUM	SYMPTOMS / NOTES
BREAKFAST				
SNACK				
LUNCH				
SNACK				
DINNER				
	DAILY SODIUM TOTAL			

NOTES :

SODIUM TRACKER

DAILY SODIUM INTAKE GOAL :

DATE :

	FOOD & DRINKS	SERVING SIZE	SODIUM	SYMPTOMS / NOTES
BREAKFAST				
SNACK				
LUNCH				
SNACK				
DINNER				
	DAILY SODIUM TOTAL			

NOTES :

SODIUM TRACKER

DAILY SODIUM INTAKE GOAL :

DATE :

	FOOD & DRINKS	SERVING SIZE	SODIUM	SYMPTOMS / NOTES
BREAKFAST				
SNACK				
LUNCH				
SNACK				
DINNER				
	DAILY SODIUM TOTAL			

NOTES :

SODIUM TRACKER

DAILY SODIUM INTAKE GOAL :	DATE :

	FOOD & DRINKS	SERVING SIZE	SODIUM	SYMPTOMS / NOTES
BREAKFAST				
SNACK				
LUNCH				
SNACK				
DINNER				
	DAILY SODIUM TOTAL			

NOTES :

SODIUM TRACKER

DAILY SODIUM INTAKE GOAL :

DATE :

	FOOD & DRINKS	SERVING SIZE	SODIUM	SYMPTOMS / NOTES
BREAKFAST				
SNACK				
LUNCH				
SNACK				
DINNER				
	DAILY SODIUM TOTAL			

NOTES :

SODIUM TRACKER

DAILY SODIUM INTAKE GOAL :

DATE :

	FOOD & DRINKS	SERVING SIZE	SODIUM	SYMPTOMS / NOTES
BREAKFAST				
SNACK				
LUNCH				
SNACK				
DINNER				
	DAILY SODIUM TOTAL			

NOTES :

SODIUM TRACKER

DAILY SODIUM INTAKE GOAL :

DATE :

	FOOD & DRINKS	SERVING SIZE	SODIUM	SYMPTOMS / NOTES
BREAKFAST				
SNACK				
LUNCH				
SNACK				
DINNER				
	DAILY SODIUM TOTAL			

NOTES :

SODIUM TRACKER

DAILY SODIUM INTAKE GOAL :

DATE :

	FOOD & DRINKS	SERVING SIZE	SODIUM	SYMPTOMS / NOTES
BREAKFAST				
SNACK				
LUNCH				
SNACK				
DINNER				
	DAILY SODIUM TOTAL			

NOTES :

SODIUM TRACKER

DAILY SODIUM INTAKE GOAL :

DATE :

	FOOD & DRINKS	SERVING SIZE	SODIUM	SYMPTOMS / NOTES
BREAKFAST				
SNACK				
LUNCH				
SNACK				
DINNER				
	DAILY SODIUM TOTAL			

NOTES :

SODIUM TRACKER

DAILY SODIUM INTAKE GOAL :

DATE :

	FOOD & DRINKS	SERVING SIZE	SODIUM	SYMPTOMS / NOTES
BREAKFAST				
SNACK				
LUNCH				
SNACK				
DINNER				
	DAILY SODIUM TOTAL			

NOTES :

SODIUM TRACKER

DAILY SODIUM INTAKE GOAL :

DATE :

	FOOD & DRINKS	SERVING SIZE	SODIUM	SYMPTOMS / NOTES
BREAKFAST				
SNACK				
LUNCH				
SNACK				
DINNER				
	DAILY SODIUM TOTAL			

NOTES :

SODIUM TRACKER

DAILY SODIUM INTAKE GOAL :

DATE :

	FOOD & DRINKS	SERVING SIZE	SODIUM	SYMPTOMS / NOTES
BREAKFAST				
SNACK				
LUNCH				
SNACK				
DINNER				
	DAILY SODIUM TOTAL			

NOTES :

SODIUM TRACKER

DAILY SODIUM INTAKE GOAL :

DATE :

	FOOD & DRINKS	SERVING SIZE	SODIUM	SYMPTOMS / NOTES
BREAKFAST				
SNACK				
LUNCH				
SNACK				
DINNER				
	DAILY SODIUM TOTAL			

NOTES :

SODIUM TRACKER

DAILY SODIUM INTAKE GOAL :

DATE :

	FOOD & DRINKS	SERVING SIZE	SODIUM	SYMPTOMS / NOTES
BREAKFAST				
SNACK				
LUNCH				
SNACK				
DINNER				
	DAILY SODIUM TOTAL			

NOTES :

SODIUM TRACKER

DAILY SODIUM INTAKE GOAL :

DATE :

	FOOD & DRINKS	SERVING SIZE	SODIUM	SYMPTOMS / NOTES
BREAKFAST				
SNACK				
LUNCH				
SNACK				
DINNER				
	DAILY SODIUM TOTAL			

NOTES :

SODIUM TRACKER

DAILY SODIUM INTAKE GOAL :

DATE :

	FOOD & DRINKS	SERVING SIZE	SODIUM	SYMPTOMS / NOTES
BREAKFAST				
SNACK				
LUNCH				
SNACK				
DINNER				
	DAILY SODIUM TOTAL			

NOTES :

SODIUM TRACKER

DAILY SODIUM INTAKE GOAL :

DATE :

	FOOD & DRINKS	SERVING SIZE	SODIUM	SYMPTOMS / NOTES
BREAKFAST				
SNACK				
LUNCH				
SNACK				
DINNER				
	DAILY SODIUM TOTAL			

NOTES :

SODIUM TRACKER

DAILY SODIUM INTAKE GOAL :

DATE :

	FOOD & DRINKS	SERVING SIZE	SODIUM	SYMPTOMS / NOTES
BREAKFAST				
SNACK				
LUNCH				
SNACK				
DINNER				
	DAILY SODIUM TOTAL			

NOTES :

SODIUM TRACKER

DAILY SODIUM INTAKE GOAL :

DATE :

	FOOD & DRINKS	SERVING SIZE	SODIUM	SYMPTOMS / NOTES
BREAKFAST				
SNACK				
LUNCH				
SNACK				
DINNER				
	DAILY SODIUM TOTAL			

NOTES :

SODIUM TRACKER

DAILY SODIUM INTAKE GOAL :

DATE :

	FOOD & DRINKS	SERVING SIZE	SODIUM	SYMPTOMS / NOTES
BREAKFAST				
SNACK				
LUNCH				
SNACK				
DINNER				
	DAILY SODIUM TOTAL			

NOTES :

SODIUM TRACKER

DAILY SODIUM INTAKE GOAL :

DATE :

	FOOD & DRINKS	SERVING SIZE	SODIUM	SYMPTOMS / NOTES
BREAKFAST				
SNACK				
LUNCH				
SNACK				
DINNER				
	DAILY SODIUM TOTAL			

NOTES :

SODIUM TRACKER

DAILY SODIUM INTAKE GOAL :

DATE :

	FOOD & DRINKS	SERVING SIZE	SODIUM	SYMPTOMS / NOTES
BREAKFAST				
SNACK				
LUNCH				
SNACK				
DINNER				
	DAILY SODIUM TOTAL			

NOTES :

SODIUM TRACKER

DAILY SODIUM INTAKE GOAL :

DATE :

	FOOD & DRINKS	SERVING SIZE	SODIUM	SYMPTOMS / NOTES
BREAKFAST				
SNACK				
LUNCH				
SNACK				
DINNER				
	DAILY SODIUM TOTAL			

NOTES :

SODIUM TRACKER

DAILY SODIUM INTAKE GOAL :

DATE :

	FOOD & DRINKS	SERVING SIZE	SODIUM	SYMPTOMS / NOTES
BREAKFAST				
SNACK				
LUNCH				
SNACK				
DINNER				
	DAILY SODIUM TOTAL			

NOTES :

SODIUM TRACKER

DAILY SODIUM INTAKE GOAL :

DATE :

	FOOD & DRINKS	SERVING SIZE	SODIUM	SYMPTOMS / NOTES
BREAKFAST				
SNACK				
LUNCH				
SNACK				
DINNER				
	DAILY SODIUM TOTAL			

NOTES :

SODIUM TRACKER

DAILY SODIUM INTAKE GOAL :

DATE :

	FOOD & DRINKS	SERVING SIZE	SODIUM	SYMPTOMS / NOTES
BREAKFAST				
SNACK				
LUNCH				
SNACK				
DINNER				
	DAILY SODIUM TOTAL			

NOTES :

SODIUM TRACKER

DAILY SODIUM INTAKE GOAL :

DATE :

	FOOD & DRINKS	SERVING SIZE	SODIUM	SYMPTOMS / NOTES
BREAKFAST				
SNACK				
LUNCH				
SNACK				
DINNER				
	DAILY SODIUM TOTAL			

NOTES :

SODIUM TRACKER

DAILY SODIUM INTAKE GOAL :

DATE :

	FOOD & DRINKS	SERVING SIZE	SODIUM	SYMPTOMS / NOTES
BREAKFAST				
SNACK				
LUNCH				
SNACK				
DINNER				
	DAILY SODIUM TOTAL			

NOTES :

SODIUM TRACKER

DAILY SODIUM INTAKE GOAL :

DATE :

	FOOD & DRINKS	SERVING SIZE	SODIUM	SYMPTOMS / NOTES
BREAKFAST				
SNACK				
LUNCH				
SNACK				
DINNER				
	DAILY SODIUM TOTAL			

NOTES :

SODIUM TRACKER

DAILY SODIUM INTAKE GOAL :

DATE :

	FOOD & DRINKS	SERVING SIZE	SODIUM	SYMPTOMS / NOTES
BREAKFAST				
SNACK				
LUNCH				
SNACK				
DINNER				
	DAILY SODIUM TOTAL			

NOTES :

SODIUM TRACKER

DAILY SODIUM INTAKE GOAL :

DATE :

	FOOD & DRINKS	SERVING SIZE	SODIUM	SYMPTOMS / NOTES
BREAKFAST				
SNACK				
LUNCH				
SNACK				
DINNER				
	DAILY SODIUM TOTAL			

NOTES :

SODIUM TRACKER

DAILY SODIUM INTAKE GOAL :

DATE :

	FOOD & DRINKS	SERVING SIZE	SODIUM	SYMPTOMS / NOTES
BREAKFAST				
SNACK				
LUNCH				
SNACK				
DINNER				
	DAILY SODIUM TOTAL			

NOTES :

SODIUM TRACKER

DAILY SODIUM INTAKE GOAL :

DATE :

	FOOD & DRINKS	SERVING SIZE	SODIUM	SYMPTOMS / NOTES
BREAKFAST				
SNACK				
LUNCH				
SNACK				
DINNER				
	DAILY SODIUM TOTAL			

NOTES :

SODIUM TRACKER

DAILY SODIUM INTAKE GOAL :

DATE :

	FOOD & DRINKS	SERVING SIZE	SODIUM	SYMPTOMS / NOTES
BREAKFAST				
SNACK				
LUNCH				
SNACK				
DINNER				
	DAILY SODIUM TOTAL			

NOTES :

SODIUM TRACKER

DAILY SODIUM INTAKE GOAL :

DATE :

	FOOD & DRINKS	SERVING SIZE	SODIUM	SYMPTOMS / NOTES
BREAKFAST				
SNACK				
LUNCH				
SNACK				
DINNER				
	DAILY SODIUM TOTAL			

NOTES :

SODIUM TRACKER

DAILY SODIUM INTAKE GOAL :

DATE :

	FOOD & DRINKS	SERVING SIZE	SODIUM	SYMPTOMS / NOTES
BREAKFAST				
SNACK				
LUNCH				
SNACK				
DINNER				
	DAILY SODIUM TOTAL			

NOTES :

SODIUM TRACKER

DAILY SODIUM INTAKE GOAL :

DATE :

	FOOD & DRINKS	SERVING SIZE	SODIUM	SYMPTOMS / NOTES
BREAKFAST				
SNACK				
LUNCH				
SNACK				
DINNER				
	DAILY SODIUM TOTAL			

NOTES :

SODIUM TRACKER

DAILY SODIUM INTAKE GOAL :

DATE :

	FOOD & DRINKS	SERVING SIZE	SODIUM	SYMPTOMS / NOTES
BREAKFAST				
SNACK				
LUNCH				
SNACK				
DINNER				
	DAILY SODIUM TOTAL			

NOTES :

SODIUM TRACKER

DAILY SODIUM INTAKE GOAL :	DATE :

	FOOD & DRINKS	SERVING SIZE	SODIUM	SYMPTOMS / NOTES
BREAKFAST				
SNACK				
LUNCH				
SNACK				
DINNER				
	DAILY SODIUM TOTAL			

NOTES :

SODIUM TRACKER

DAILY SODIUM INTAKE GOAL :

DATE :

	FOOD & DRINKS	SERVING SIZE	SODIUM	SYMPTOMS / NOTES
BREAKFAST				
SNACK				
LUNCH				
SNACK				
DINNER				
	DAILY SODIUM TOTAL			

NOTES :

SODIUM TRACKER

DAILY SODIUM INTAKE GOAL :

DATE :

	FOOD & DRINKS	SERVING SIZE	SODIUM	SYMPTOMS / NOTES
BREAKFAST				
SNACK				
LUNCH				
SNACK				
DINNER				
	DAILY SODIUM TOTAL			

NOTES :

SODIUM TRACKER

DAILY SODIUM INTAKE GOAL :

DATE :

	FOOD & DRINKS	SERVING SIZE	SODIUM	SYMPTOMS / NOTES
BREAKFAST				
SNACK				
LUNCH				
SNACK				
DINNER				
	DAILY SODIUM TOTAL			

NOTES :

SODIUM TRACKER

DAILY SODIUM INTAKE GOAL :

DATE :

	FOOD & DRINKS	SERVING SIZE	SODIUM	SYMPTOMS / NOTES
BREAKFAST				
SNACK				
LUNCH				
SNACK				
DINNER				
	DAILY SODIUM TOTAL			

NOTES :

SODIUM TRACKER

DAILY SODIUM INTAKE GOAL :

DATE :

	FOOD & DRINKS	SERVING SIZE	SODIUM	SYMPTOMS / NOTES
BREAKFAST				
SNACK				
LUNCH				
SNACK				
DINNER				
	DAILY SODIUM TOTAL			

NOTES :

SODIUM TRACKER

DAILY SODIUM INTAKE GOAL :

DATE :

	FOOD & DRINKS	SERVING SIZE	SODIUM	SYMPTOMS / NOTES
BREAKFAST				
SNACK				
LUNCH				
SNACK				
DINNER				
	DAILY SODIUM TOTAL			

NOTES :

SODIUM TRACKER

DAILY SODIUM INTAKE GOAL :

DATE :

	FOOD & DRINKS	SERVING SIZE	SODIUM	SYMPTOMS / NOTES
BREAKFAST				
SNACK				
LUNCH				
SNACK				
DINNER				
	DAILY SODIUM TOTAL			

NOTES :

SODIUM TRACKER

DAILY SODIUM INTAKE GOAL :

DATE :

	FOOD & DRINKS	SERVING SIZE	SODIUM	SYMPTOMS / NOTES
BREAKFAST				
SNACK				
LUNCH				
SNACK				
DINNER				
	DAILY SODIUM TOTAL			

NOTES :

SODIUM TRACKER

DAILY SODIUM INTAKE GOAL :

DATE :

	FOOD & DRINKS	SERVING SIZE	SODIUM	SYMPTOMS / NOTES
BREAKFAST				
SNACK				
LUNCH				
SNACK				
DINNER				
	DAILY SODIUM TOTAL			

NOTES :

SODIUM TRACKER

DAILY SODIUM INTAKE GOAL :

DATE :

	FOOD & DRINKS	SERVING SIZE	SODIUM	SYMPTOMS / NOTES
BREAKFAST				
SNACK				
LUNCH				
SNACK				
DINNER				
	DAILY SODIUM TOTAL			

NOTES :

SODIUM TRACKER

DAILY SODIUM INTAKE GOAL :

DATE :

	FOOD & DRINKS	SERVING SIZE	SODIUM	SYMPTOMS / NOTES
BREAKFAST				
SNACK				
LUNCH				
SNACK				
DINNER				
	DAILY SODIUM TOTAL			

NOTES :

SODIUM TRACKER

DAILY SODIUM INTAKE GOAL :

DATE :

	FOOD & DRINKS	SERVING SIZE	SODIUM	SYMPTOMS / NOTES
BREAKFAST				
SNACK				
LUNCH				
SNACK				
DINNER				
	DAILY SODIUM TOTAL			

NOTES :

SODIUM TRACKER

DAILY SODIUM INTAKE GOAL :

DATE :

	FOOD & DRINKS	SERVING SIZE	SODIUM	SYMPTOMS / NOTES
BREAKFAST				
SNACK				
LUNCH				
SNACK				
DINNER				
	DAILY SODIUM TOTAL			

NOTES :

SODIUM TRACKER

DAILY SODIUM INTAKE GOAL :

DATE :

	FOOD & DRINKS	SERVING SIZE	SODIUM	SYMPTOMS / NOTES
BREAKFAST				
SNACK				
LUNCH				
SNACK				
DINNER				
	DAILY SODIUM TOTAL			

NOTES :

SODIUM TRACKER

DAILY SODIUM INTAKE GOAL :

DATE :

	FOOD & DRINKS	SERVING SIZE	SODIUM	SYMPTOMS / NOTES
BREAKFAST				
SNACK				
LUNCH				
SNACK				
DINNER				
	DAILY SODIUM TOTAL			

NOTES :

SODIUM TRACKER

DAILY SODIUM INTAKE GOAL :

DATE :

	FOOD & DRINKS	SERVING SIZE	SODIUM	SYMPTOMS / NOTES
BREAKFAST				
SNACK				
LUNCH				
SNACK				
DINNER				
	DAILY SODIUM TOTAL			

NOTES :

SODIUM TRACKER

DAILY SODIUM INTAKE GOAL :

DATE :

	FOOD & DRINKS	SERVING SIZE	SODIUM	SYMPTOMS / NOTES
BREAKFAST				
SNACK				
LUNCH				
SNACK				
DINNER				
	DAILY SODIUM TOTAL			

NOTES :

SODIUM TRACKER

DAILY SODIUM INTAKE GOAL :	DATE :

	FOOD & DRINKS	SERVING SIZE	SODIUM	SYMPTOMS / NOTES
BREAKFAST				
SNACK				
LUNCH				
SNACK				
DINNER				
	DAILY SODIUM TOTAL			

NOTES :

SODIUM TRACKER

DAILY SODIUM INTAKE GOAL :

DATE :

	FOOD & DRINKS	SERVING SIZE	SODIUM	SYMPTOMS / NOTES
BREAKFAST				
SNACK				
LUNCH				
SNACK				
DINNER				
	DAILY SODIUM TOTAL			

NOTES :

SODIUM TRACKER

DAILY SODIUM INTAKE GOAL :

DATE :

	FOOD & DRINKS	SERVING SIZE	SODIUM	SYMPTOMS / NOTES
BREAKFAST				
SNACK				
LUNCH				
SNACK				
DINNER				
	DAILY SODIUM TOTAL			

NOTES :

SODIUM TRACKER

DAILY SODIUM INTAKE GOAL :

DATE :

	FOOD & DRINKS	SERVING SIZE	SODIUM	SYMPTOMS / NOTES
BREAKFAST				
SNACK				
LUNCH				
SNACK				
DINNER				
	DAILY SODIUM TOTAL			

NOTES :

SODIUM TRACKER

DAILY SODIUM INTAKE GOAL :

DATE :

	FOOD & DRINKS	SERVING SIZE	SODIUM	SYMPTOMS / NOTES
BREAKFAST				
SNACK				
LUNCH				
SNACK				
DINNER				
	DAILY SODIUM TOTAL			

NOTES :

SODIUM TRACKER

DAILY SODIUM INTAKE GOAL :

DATE :

	FOOD & DRINKS	SERVING SIZE	SODIUM	SYMPTOMS / NOTES
BREAKFAST				
SNACK				
LUNCH				
SNACK				
DINNER				
	DAILY SODIUM TOTAL			

NOTES :

SODIUM TRACKER

DAILY SODIUM INTAKE GOAL :

DATE :

	FOOD & DRINKS	SERVING SIZE	SODIUM	SYMPTOMS / NOTES
BREAKFAST				
SNACK				
LUNCH				
SNACK				
DINNER				
	DAILY SODIUM TOTAL			

NOTES :

SODIUM TRACKER

DAILY SODIUM INTAKE GOAL :

DATE :

	FOOD & DRINKS	SERVING SIZE	SODIUM	SYMPTOMS / NOTES
BREAKFAST				
SNACK				
LUNCH				
SNACK				
DINNER				
	DAILY SODIUM TOTAL			

NOTES :

SODIUM TRACKER

DAILY SODIUM INTAKE GOAL :

DATE :

	FOOD & DRINKS	SERVING SIZE	SODIUM	SYMPTOMS / NOTES
BREAKFAST				
SNACK				
LUNCH				
SNACK				
DINNER				
	DAILY SODIUM TOTAL			

NOTES :

SODIUM TRACKER

DAILY SODIUM INTAKE GOAL :

DATE :

	FOOD & DRINKS	SERVING SIZE	SODIUM	SYMPTOMS / NOTES
BREAKFAST				
SNACK				
LUNCH				
SNACK				
DINNER				
	DAILY SODIUM TOTAL			

NOTES :

SODIUM TRACKER

DAILY SODIUM INTAKE GOAL :

DATE :

	FOOD & DRINKS	SERVING SIZE	SODIUM	SYMPTOMS / NOTES
BREAKFAST				
SNACK				
LUNCH				
SNACK				
DINNER				
	DAILY SODIUM TOTAL			

NOTES :

SODIUM TRACKER

DAILY SODIUM INTAKE GOAL :

DATE :

	FOOD & DRINKS	SERVING SIZE	SODIUM	SYMPTOMS / NOTES
BREAKFAST				
SNACK				
LUNCH				
SNACK				
DINNER				
	DAILY SODIUM TOTAL			

NOTES :

SODIUM TRACKER

DAILY SODIUM INTAKE GOAL :

DATE :

	FOOD & DRINKS	SERVING SIZE	SODIUM	SYMPTOMS / NOTES
BREAKFAST				
SNACK				
LUNCH				
SNACK				
DINNER				
	DAILY SODIUM TOTAL			

NOTES :

SODIUM TRACKER

DAILY SODIUM INTAKE GOAL :

DATE :

	FOOD & DRINKS	SERVING SIZE	SODIUM	SYMPTOMS / NOTES
BREAKFAST				
SNACK				
LUNCH				
SNACK				
DINNER				
	DAILY SODIUM TOTAL			

NOTES :

SODIUM TRACKER

DAILY SODIUM INTAKE GOAL :

DATE :

	FOOD & DRINKS	SERVING SIZE	SODIUM	SYMPTOMS / NOTES
BREAKFAST				
SNACK				
LUNCH				
SNACK				
DINNER				
	DAILY SODIUM TOTAL			

NOTES :

SODIUM TRACKER

DAILY SODIUM INTAKE GOAL :

DATE :

	FOOD & DRINKS	SERVING SIZE	SODIUM	SYMPTOMS / NOTES
BREAKFAST				
SNACK				
LUNCH				
SNACK				
DINNER				
	DAILY SODIUM TOTAL			

NOTES :

SODIUM TRACKER

DAILY SODIUM INTAKE GOAL :

DATE :

	FOOD & DRINKS	SERVING SIZE	SODIUM	SYMPTOMS / NOTES
BREAKFAST				
SNACK				
LUNCH				
SNACK				
DINNER				
	DAILY SODIUM TOTAL			

NOTES :

Made in the USA
Monee, IL
28 May 2023